THE SWEET LIFE WITH DIABETES: BALANCING HEALTH AND HAPPINESS

DIPAN KUMAR DAS
SUDIP KUMAR DAS

This book is dedicated to all the individuals and families affected by diabetes. Your perseverance, resilience, and dedication to managing this condition is an inspiration to us all. May this book provide you with valuable information, tools, and resources to help you navigate the challenges of diabetes and lead a healthy, fulfilling life.

Foreword

Living with diabetes can be challenging, but it doesn't have to be a barrier to living a full and happy life. With the right knowledge, tools, and support, people with diabetes can manage their condition and thrive.

In this book, you'll find a comprehensive guide to managing diabetes, from understanding the condition and its causes to making healthy lifestyle choices, managing medications and medical appointments, and coping with the emotional impact of diabetes.

As someone who has seen the impact of diabetes on loved ones, I know how important it is to have access to accurate and helpful information. This book is an excellent resource for anyone living with diabetes, their family members, and healthcare providers.

I encourage you to take control of your diabetes and use the information in this book to live a healthy, fulfilling life. Remember, you're not alone on this journey. With the right support, you can thrive with diabetes.

Preface

Living with diabetes can be challenging, but it doesn't have to be a barrier to leading a happy, healthy, and fulfilling life. With the right information, tools, and support, people with diabetes can manage their condition and prevent or delay complications. That's why I wrote this book, to provide a comprehensive guide to managing diabetes through nutrition, exercise, medication, and lifestyle changes.

As a healthcare professional with many years of experience working with people with diabetes, I have seen firsthand the impact that effective diabetes management can have on a person's health and wellbeing. I have also seen the consequences of poorly managed diabetes, such as kidney disease, nerve damage, and blindness, which can be devastating for individuals and families.

The good news is that with the right knowledge and support, people with diabetes can take control of their condition and reduce their risk of complications. This book covers everything you need to know about managing diabetes, from understanding the basics of blood sugar control to developing healthy eating habits, staying physically active, coping with the emotional impact of diabetes, and managing medications and medical appointments.

I hope this book will be a valuable resource for anyone living with diabetes or caring for someone with diabetes. By working together, we can all take steps towards better diabetes management and a healthier future.

Prologue

As I sat in my doctor's office and heard the words "You have diabetes," I felt a wave of fear wash over me. I knew very little about the condition, and my mind was flooded with questions and concerns. How would this affect my daily life? What kind of changes would I need to make to my diet and exercise routine? How would I manage my medications and doctor's appointments?

Over time, I learned that living with diabetes is a journey, and it requires patience, dedication, and a willingness to learn. I also learned that with the right tools and resources, it is possible to manage diabetes and live a healthy, fulfilling life.

In writing this book, I hope to provide those tools and resources to others who are facing a similar journey. Whether you have just been diagnosed with diabetes, or you have been living with the condition for years, this book is designed to be a comprehensive guide to managing diabetes through nutrition, exercise, medication, and emotional support.

My goal is to empower you with the knowledge and skills you need to take control of your diabetes and live your life to the fullest. I believe that with the right mindset and the right support, anything is possible. So let's begin this journey together, one step at a time.

1

What is Diabetes?

- **Definition of diabetes**

Diabetes is a chronic medical condition characterized by high levels of glucose (sugar) in the blood. It occurs when the body is unable to produce or properly use insulin, a hormone that regulates blood sugar levels. As a result, people with diabetes may experience a range of symptoms and health complications, including fatigue, frequent urination, excessive thirst, blurred vision, nerve damage, and cardiovascular disease. There are several types of diabetes, including Type 1, Type 2, gestational diabetes, and prediabetes. Each type has its own causes, symptoms, and treatment options.

- **Types of diabetes (Type 1, Type 2, gestational diabetes, prediabetes)**

There are four main types of diabetes:

Type 1 diabetes: Type 1 diabetes is an autoimmune disease in which the body's immune system attacks and destroys the insulin-producing cells in the pancreas. As a result, the body is unable to produce enough insulin to regulate blood sugar levels. Type 1 diabetes usually develops in childhood or adolescence, but can also occur in adults.

Type 2 diabetes: Type 2 diabetes is the most common form of diabetes, accounting for around 90% of all cases. It occurs when the body becomes resistant to the effects of insulin, or when the pancreas is unable to produce enough insulin to meet the body's needs. Type 2 diabetes is typically associated with lifestyle factors such as obesity, lack of exercise, and poor diet.

Gestational diabetes: Gestational diabetes is a type of diabetes that develops during pregnancy. It occurs when the body is unable to produce enough insulin to meet the increased demands of pregnancy. Gestational diabetes usually resolves after childbirth, but women who have had gestational diabetes are at increased risk of developing Type 2 diabetes later in life.

Prediabetes: Prediabetes is a condition in which blood sugar levels are higher than normal but not yet high enough to be classified as Type 2 diabetes. Prediabetes is often a precursor to Type 2 diabetes and can be reversed with lifestyle changes such as diet and exercise. People with prediabetes are also at increased risk of developing heart disease and other health complications.

- **Causes and risk factors**

The causes of diabetes vary depending on the type of diabetes.

For Type 1 diabetes, the exact cause is unknown, but it is believed to be an autoimmune disorder in which the body's immune system mistakenly attacks and destroys the insulin-producing cells in the pancreas.

For Type 2 diabetes, the causes are complex and multifactorial, involving a combination of genetic and lifestyle factors. Some of the risk factors associated with Type 2 diabetes include:

Obesity or being overweight

Lack of physical activity

Unhealthy diet, particularly one high in sugar and refined carbohydrates

Family history of diabetes

Age (the risk of Type 2 diabetes increases with age)

Race or ethnicity (people of certain racial or ethnic groups, such as African Americans, Hispanic/Latino Americans, and Native Americans, are at higher risk of developing Type 2 diabetes)

Gestational diabetes is thought to be caused by a combination of hormonal and genetic factors. Women who are overweight or have a family history of diabetes are at increased risk of developing gestational diabetes.

Prediabetes is often a result of the same risk factors as Type 2 diabetes, including obesity, unhealthy diet, and lack of physical activity. However, some people may develop prediabetes due to genetic factors or other underlying medical conditions.

- **Symptoms and warning signs**

The symptoms and warning signs of diabetes vary depending on the type of diabetes, and some people may not experience any symptoms at all. However, some common symptoms and warning signs to look out for include:

Type 1 diabetes:
Frequent urination
Increased thirst
Extreme hunger
Unintended weight loss
Fatigue and weakness
Blurred vision
Slow-healing sores or frequent infections
Type 2 diabetes:
Any of the symptoms of Type 1 diabetes
Tingling, pain, or numbness in the hands or feet
Recurrent infections or slow-healing sores
Areas of darkened skin, particularly around the neck, armpits, and groin
Increased hunger, even after eating
Erectile dysfunction in men
Gestational diabetes:

Any of the symptoms of Type 2 diabetes

Excessive weight gain during pregnancy

Large baby at birth (over 9 pounds)

High blood pressure during pregnancy

Family history of Type 2 diabetes or gestational diabetes

Prediabetes:

No symptoms may be present

Some people may experience symptoms similar to those of Type 2 diabetes, such as increased thirst and frequent urination

It is important to note that many of these symptoms can be mild and may be easily overlooked or attributed to other causes. If you experience any of these symptoms or are at increased risk for diabetes, it is important to talk to your doctor and get tested for diabetes. Early diagnosis and treatment can help prevent or delay the onset of diabetes-related complications.

2

Diagnosing Diabetes

- **Blood tests used to diagnose diabetes (Fasting plasma glucose, Oral glucose tolerance test, Hemoglobin A1C test)**

Diabetes is typically diagnosed through blood tests that measure glucose levels in the bloodstream. There are several different tests that can be used to diagnose diabetes, including:

1. Fasting plasma glucose (FPG) test: This test measures your blood sugar level after an overnight fast of at least 8 hours. A blood sample is taken and analyzed to determine your glucose level. A result of 126 mg/dL (7.0 mmol/L) or higher on two separate occasions indicates a diagnosis of diabetes.
2. Oral glucose tolerance test (OGTT): This test is performed after an overnight fast, and involves drinking a sugary solution. Blood samples are taken before and 2 hours after drinking the solution to measure how well your body processes glucose. A result of 200 mg/dL (11.1 mmol/L) or higher after 2 hours indicates a diagnosis of diabetes.
3. Hemoglobin A1C (HbA1C) test: This test measures your average blood sugar levels over the past 2-3 months by analyzing the percentage of glucose that is attached to hemoglobin molecules in your red blood cells. A result of 6.5% or higher on two separate occasions indicates a diagnosis of diabetes.

In addition to these tests, your doctor may also perform additional tests to rule out other conditions that can cause similar symptoms to diabetes, such as thyroid disorders and pancreatitis.

It is important to note that diabetes is a progressive disease, and early diagnosis and treatment can help prevent or delay the onset of complications. If you have any risk factors for diabetes or are experiencing symptoms, it is important to talk to your doctor and get tested. Regular check-ups and blood tests can help detect diabetes early and prevent long-term complications.

It is also worth noting that the American Diabetes Association recommends that all adults over the age of 45 should be tested for diabetes every three years, regardless of whether they have any risk factors or symptoms.

For individuals who are at higher risk for diabetes, such as those with a family history of the disease or who are overweight or obese, more frequent testing may be recommended. Women who have had gestational diabetes during pregnancy are also at increased risk of developing Type 2 diabetes and should be tested regularly.

It is important to follow your doctor's instructions when preparing for a diabetes test, as some tests require you to fast for a certain amount of time before the test. It is also important to inform your doctor of any medications you are taking, as some medications can affect your blood sugar levels and may need to be adjusted before the test.

Early diagnosis and treatment of diabetes can help prevent or delay the onset of serious complications, such as heart disease, stroke, kidney disease, nerve damage, and vision loss. If you are diagnosed with diabetes, it is important to work closely with your healthcare team to develop a personalized treatment plan that includes a healthy diet, regular exercise, and appropriate medication or insulin therapy. Regular blood sugar monitoring and check-ups are also important to help manage your diabetes and prevent long-term complications.

In addition to the blood tests mentioned earlier, there are other ways to diagnose diabetes, such as random plasma glucose tests, which measure blood sugar levels at any time of the day regardless of when the person last ate. However, this method is not as reliable as the other diagnostic tests mentioned earlier and is not usually used to confirm a diagnosis of diabetes.

It is important to note that a diagnosis of diabetes does not mean that your life is over or that you cannot lead a healthy, fulfilling life. With proper management and treatment, many people with diabetes are able to live long, healthy lives. It is important to work closely with your healthcare team to manage your diabetes and make healthy lifestyle choices to help prevent or delay the onset of complications.

If you have been diagnosed with diabetes, it is important to monitor your blood sugar levels regularly and follow your doctor's recommendations for managing your condition. This may include checking your blood sugar levels at home with a glucose meter, taking medication or insulin as prescribed, making dietary changes, and getting regular exercise.

Managing diabetes can be challenging, but with the right support and resources, it is possible to lead a healthy, active life. Many organizations, such as the American Diabetes Association, offer resources and support for people with diabetes and their families. It is important to take advantage of these resources and reach out for help when needed.

In the next chapter, we will discuss the different treatment options available for diabetes and how to develop a personalized treatment plan with your healthcare team.

- Interpreting blood test results

When you receive your blood test results, it's important to understand what they mean and what your numbers indicate about your diabetes. The following are some key numbers to look for and their interpretations:

1. Fasting plasma glucose (FPG) test: A normal FPG result is less than 100 mg/dL (5.6 mmol/L). A result between 100-125 mg/dL (5.6-6.9 mmol/L) indicates prediabetes, while a result of 126 mg/dL (7.0 mmol/L) or higher on two separate occasions indicates diabetes.

2. Oral glucose tolerance test (OGTT): A normal OGTT result is less than 140 mg/dL (7.8 mmol/L) two hours after drinking the sugary solution. A result between 140-199 mg/dL (7.8-11.0 mmol/L) indicates prediabetes, while a result of 200 mg/dL (11.1 mmol/L) or higher indicates diabetes.
3. Hemoglobin A1C (HbA1C) test: A normal HbA1C result is less than 5.7%. A result between 5.7-6.4% indicates prediabetes, while a result of 6.5% or higher on two separate occasions indicates diabetes.

It's important to note that these numbers may vary slightly depending on the laboratory and the method used to perform the test. Your healthcare provider can help interpret your results and provide personalized recommendations based on your individual situation.

In addition to these tests, your healthcare provider may also monitor your blood pressure, cholesterol levels, and kidney function to help manage your diabetes and prevent long-term complications.

Regular blood sugar monitoring at home with a glucose meter can also provide important information about how well you are managing your diabetes. Your healthcare provider can help you interpret your blood sugar readings and make adjustments to your treatment plan as needed.

Understanding your blood test results is an important part of managing your diabetes and preventing long-term complications. It is important to work closely with your healthcare provider to monitor your blood sugar levels and develop a personalized treatment plan that meets your individual needs.

- Importance of early diagnosis and treatment

Early diagnosis and treatment of diabetes are crucial for several reasons. Firstly, early diagnosis can help prevent or delay the onset of complications associated with diabetes, such as heart disease, kidney disease, nerve damage, and vision problems. The longer diabetes goes undiagnosed and untreated, the higher the risk of developing these complications.

Secondly, early treatment can help control blood sugar levels, which can reduce the risk of long-term complications. Treatment may include medication, insulin therapy, dietary changes, and exercise. With proper treatment and management, many people with diabetes are able to lead healthy, active lives.

Thirdly, early diagnosis and treatment can improve quality of life for people with diabetes. Symptoms such as excessive thirst, frequent urination, and fatigue can be debilitating and can interfere with daily activities. Treatment can help alleviate these symptoms and improve overall well-being.

In addition to the health benefits, early diagnosis and treatment of diabetes can also have financial benefits. The cost of managing diabetes can be high, but early treatment can help prevent or delay the onset of complications, which can result in significant cost savings over time.

It's important to note that even if you have already been diagnosed with diabetes, it's never too late to take steps to manage your condition and prevent or delay the onset of complications. Working closely with your healthcare team and making healthy lifestyle choices can help you achieve better health outcomes and improve your overall quality of life.

In conclusion, early diagnosis and treatment of diabetes are critical for preventing or delaying complications, improving quality of life, and reducing healthcare costs. If you suspect you may have diabetes, it's important to seek medical attention and get tested as soon as possible.

It's also important to note that some people may have diabetes without experiencing any symptoms. This is why routine blood tests are so important, especially for people who have a family history of diabetes or other risk factors.

Unfortunately, many people with diabetes remain undiagnosed for years, which can lead to serious complications. According to the Centers for Disease Control and Prevention (CDC), over 7 million Americans with diabetes are undiagnosed.

If you are at risk for diabetes or have symptoms such as frequent urination, excessive thirst, fatigue, or blurred vision, it's important to talk to your healthcare provider and get tested. The earlier diabetes is diagnosed and treated, the better the outcomes.

In addition to medical treatment, making healthy lifestyle choices can also play a significant role in managing diabetes. This includes eating a healthy diet, exercising regularly, maintaining a healthy weight, and not smoking. These lifestyle changes can help control blood sugar levels, reduce the risk of complications, and improve overall health and well-being.

In summary, early diagnosis and treatment of diabetes are crucial for preventing complications, improving quality of life, and reducing healthcare costs. If you are at risk for diabetes or have symptoms, don't wait to get tested. Talk to your healthcare provider and take steps to manage your condition and live a healthy, active life.

3

Monitoring Blood Sugar

- **The importance of monitoring blood sugar levels**

Monitoring blood sugar levels is a critical part of managing diabetes. It allows people with diabetes to understand how their body responds to different foods, activities, and medications, and helps them make informed decisions about managing their condition.

Consistently high blood sugar levels can lead to serious complications, such as heart disease, kidney damage, nerve damage, and vision problems. On the other hand, low blood sugar levels can cause symptoms such as shakiness, confusion, and even loss of consciousness.

By monitoring blood sugar levels regularly, people with diabetes can identify patterns and trends in their blood sugar levels and make adjustments to their treatment plan as needed. This can help prevent complications and improve overall health outcomes.

Blood sugar monitoring can be done using a variety of methods, including fingerstick testing, continuous glucose monitoring (CGM), and flash glucose monitoring. The method used will depend on individual preferences and healthcare provider recommendations.

For people with type 1 diabetes, monitoring blood sugar levels is especially important, as they require insulin therapy to manage their condition. For people with type 2 diabetes, monitoring blood sugar levels may also be necessary, especially if they are taking medications that lower blood sugar levels.

In summary, monitoring blood sugar levels is a critical part of managing diabetes and preventing complications. It allows people with diabetes to make informed decisions about their treatment plan and take control of their health. If you have diabetes, talk to your healthcare provider about the best method of blood sugar monitoring for you.

- **Methods of blood sugar monitoring (self-monitoring, continuous glucose monitoring)**

There are several methods of blood sugar monitoring available to people with diabetes. The most common methods include self-monitoring of blood glucose (SMBG) and continuous glucose monitoring (CGM).

1. Self-monitoring of blood glucose (SMBG): SMBG involves checking blood sugar levels using a glucose meter and test strips. This method requires a small blood sample obtained through a finger prick. The test results can provide a snapshot of blood

sugar levels at a particular point in time. This method is generally recommended for people with type 1 diabetes who require insulin therapy and for people with type 2 diabetes who are on medications that lower blood sugar levels.

2. Continuous glucose monitoring (CGM): CGM uses a small sensor that is inserted under the skin to measure glucose levels in the interstitial fluid (fluid between cells). The sensor is connected to a transmitter that sends real-time glucose readings to a receiver or smartphone app. This method provides a continuous stream of glucose data, allowing people with diabetes to monitor their blood sugar levels throughout the day and night. CGM is often recommended for people with type 1 diabetes who require intensive insulin therapy, but can also be helpful for people with type 2 diabetes who are on multiple medications.

3. Flash glucose monitoring: Flash glucose monitoring is a newer method of blood sugar monitoring that involves a sensor worn on the back of the upper arm. The

sensor measures glucose levels in the interstitial fluid and can be scanned with a smartphone to obtain glucose readings. This method provides similar benefits to CGM, such as continuous glucose data, but without the need for a transmitter or receiver.

4. Urine glucose testing: Urine glucose testing involves testing urine for the presence of glucose. This method is less accurate than SMBG or CGM, as it only provides an estimate of blood sugar levels. It is not commonly used for blood sugar monitoring, but may be used in certain situations, such as for people with diabetes who are unable to perform SMBG or CGM.

5. Laboratory blood tests: Laboratory blood tests, such as the hemoglobin A1C test, can provide information about average blood sugar levels over a period of several months. This test is not used for day-to-day blood sugar monitoring, but can be used to assess long-term blood sugar control and the effectiveness of diabetes management.

Both SMBG and CGM have their own advantages and limitations. SMBG is easy to use and can provide immediate feedback on blood sugar levels, but requires regular testing throughout the day. CGM provides more comprehensive glucose data and can alert people with diabetes to highs and lows in blood sugar levels, but requires a sensor to be inserted under the skin and may not be covered by insurance.

In summary, there are several methods of blood sugar monitoring available to people with diabetes, including SMBG and CGM. Talk to your healthcare provider about the best method for you, based on your individual needs and preferences.

- **How to interpret blood sugar readings**

Interpreting blood sugar readings can be confusing, especially for people who are new to diabetes management. Here are some general guidelines for interpreting blood sugar readings:

1. Fasting blood sugar (FBS): Fasting blood sugar is a measure of blood sugar levels

after an overnight fast. Normal fasting blood sugar levels are between 70 and 99 mg/dL (3.9 to 5.5 mmol/L). Levels above 126 mg/dL (7.0 mmol/L) may indicate diabetes.

2. Postprandial blood sugar (PPBS): Postprandial blood sugar is a measure of blood sugar levels 2 hours after a meal. Normal PPBS levels are below 140 mg/dL (7.8 mmol/L). Levels above 200 mg/dL (11.1 mmol/L) may indicate diabetes.

3. Hemoglobin A1C (HbA1c): Hemoglobin A1C is a measure of average blood sugar levels over the past 2 to 3 months. Normal HbA1c levels are below 5.7%. Levels between 5.7% and 6.4% may indicate prediabetes, and levels above 6.5% may indicate diabetes.

It is important to note that blood sugar readings can vary depending on factors such as the time of day, food intake, physical activity, stress, illness, and medication use. Therefore, it is important to work with a healthcare provider to establish individualized blood sugar targets and to develop a personalized diabetes management plan. Regular blood sugar monitoring, combined with lifestyle modifications and medication management, can help prevent complications associated with diabetes.

- **Keeping blood sugar levels within a healthy range**

Keeping blood sugar levels within a healthy range is an essential part of diabetes management. Here are some tips for maintaining healthy blood sugar levels:

1. Follow a balanced diet: Eating a balanced diet that includes a variety of foods from all food groups can help regulate blood sugar levels. Choose whole grains, fruits, vegetables, lean proteins, and healthy fats. Avoid sugary drinks and foods with added sugars, as they can cause blood sugar levels to spike.
2. Monitor carbohydrate intake: Carbohydrates have the most significant impact on blood sugar levels. Monitoring carbohydrate intake and spreading out carbohydrate intake throughout the day can

help keep blood sugar levels stable. Work with a registered dietitian to develop a personalized meal plan.

3. Stay active: Regular physical activity can help improve blood sugar control by increasing insulin sensitivity. Aim for at least 150 minutes of moderate-intensity exercise per week, such as brisk walking, cycling, or swimming.

4. Take medications as prescribed: If prescribed medication for diabetes management, take them as prescribed by your healthcare provider. Skipping doses or altering the dosage can cause blood sugar levels to fluctuate.

5. Monitor blood sugar levels regularly: Monitor blood sugar levels regularly, as directed by your healthcare provider, and record the results in a logbook. Regular monitoring can help identify trends and enable adjustments to be made to diet, exercise, and medication as needed.

6. Manage stress: Stress can cause blood sugar levels to rise. Practice stress-management techniques such as meditation, deep

breathing, or yoga to help reduce stress levels.

By following these tips and working closely with a healthcare provider, it is possible to maintain healthy blood sugar levels and reduce the risk of complications associated with diabetes.

4

Understanding Carbohydrates

- **What are carbohydrates?**

Carbohydrates are one of the three macronutrients found in food, along with protein and fat. They are the body's primary source of energy and are broken down into glucose, which is used by cells as fuel. Carbohydrates are found in a variety of foods, including fruits, vegetables, grains, legumes, and dairy products.

There are two types of carbohydrates: simple and complex. Simple carbohydrates, such as table sugar, honey, and syrup, are quickly digested and can cause a rapid rise in blood sugar levels. Complex carbohydrates, such as whole grains, fruits, vegetables, and legumes, contain fiber, vitamins, and minerals, and are digested more slowly, providing sustained energy and keeping blood sugar levels stable.

It is important for people with diabetes to monitor their carbohydrate intake and choose carbohydrate sources wisely to maintain healthy blood sugar levels. Working with a registered dietitian can help develop an individualized meal plan that meets nutritional needs while managing blood sugar levels.

- **The role of carbohydrates in diabetes management**

Carbohydrates play a critical role in managing diabetes. Since carbohydrates are broken down into glucose, they have the most significant impact on blood sugar levels. Therefore, people with diabetes need to carefully monitor their carbohydrate intake to manage their blood sugar levels.

Carbohydrate counting is a common method used by people with diabetes to manage their carbohydrate intake. This involves counting the grams of carbohydrates in each meal or snack and balancing it with the amount of insulin or medication taken. By keeping track of their carbohydrate intake, people with diabetes can keep their blood sugar levels in a healthy range.

It is also essential to choose the right types of carbohydrates. As mentioned earlier, complex carbohydrates are digested more slowly and provide sustained energy, helping to keep blood sugar levels stable. In contrast, simple carbohydrates are digested quickly, leading to a rapid rise in blood sugar levels.

In summary, the role of carbohydrates in diabetes management is crucial. By monitoring carbohydrate intake, choosing the right types of carbohydrates, and working with a healthcare team, people with diabetes can effectively manage their blood sugar levels and improve their overall health.

- **Types of carbohydrates (simple vs. complex)**

There are two main types of carbohydrates: simple and complex.

1. Simple carbohydrates are made up of one or two sugar molecules and are found in foods like sugar, candy, honey, and fruit juice. These carbohydrates are digested quickly, leading to a rapid increase in blood sugar levels.
2. Complex carbohydrates, on the other hand, are made up of multiple sugar molecules and are found in foods like whole grains, vegetables, and legumes. These carbohydrates are digested more slowly, leading to a gradual increase in blood sugar levels.

It is recommended that people with diabetes choose complex carbohydrates over simple carbohydrates. Complex carbohydrates provide more sustained energy and are less likely to cause blood sugar spikes. Additionally, they are often more nutrient-dense and provide important vitamins, minerals, and fiber.

Examples of complex carbohydrates include whole grains like brown rice, quinoa, and whole wheat bread; vegetables like sweet potatoes, broccoli, and carrots; and legumes like beans, lentils, and chickpeas.

By choosing complex carbohydrates over simple carbohydrates, people with diabetes can help to manage their blood sugar levels and reduce the risk of complications.

In addition to simple and complex carbohydrates, there is another type of carbohydrate that is important to understand for diabetes management: fiber.

Fiber is a type of carbohydrate that is not digested by the body. Instead, it passes through the digestive system largely intact, providing bulk and promoting healthy bowel movements. Fiber also helps to slow the absorption of glucose into the bloodstream, which can help to prevent blood sugar spikes.

There are two types of fiber: soluble and insoluble. Soluble fiber dissolves in water and forms a gel-like substance in the digestive tract, which can help to lower cholesterol levels and improve blood sugar control. Good sources of soluble fiber include oats, barley, beans, peas, and some fruits and vegetables.

Insoluble fiber does not dissolve in water and helps to promote regular bowel movements. Good sources of insoluble fiber include whole wheat, nuts, seeds, and many fruits and vegetables.

It is recommended that people with diabetes consume a diet that is high in fiber, with a focus on whole grains, vegetables, fruits, and legumes. This can help to improve blood sugar control, promote satiety, and reduce the risk of complications such as heart disease and digestive problems.

- **How to calculate carbohydrate intake**

For people with diabetes, it is important to monitor carbohydrate intake in order to manage blood sugar levels. Here are some steps to help calculate carbohydrate intake:

1. Determine your daily carbohydrate needs: The amount of carbohydrates you need will

depend on a number of factors, including your age, weight, height, activity level, and medication use. A registered dietitian can help you determine your individual carbohydrate needs.

2. Read food labels: Most packaged foods list the total amount of carbohydrates per serving on the nutrition label. Be sure to look at the serving size as well, as this can vary from product to product.

3. Use measuring tools: Measuring cups, spoons, and food scales can help you accurately measure the amount of carbohydrates in your food.

4. Keep track of your carbohydrate intake: Whether you use a food journal, a smartphone app, or another method, keeping track of your carbohydrate intake can help you stay within your daily limits.

5. Adjust as needed: If you find that your blood sugar levels are consistently high or low, you may need to adjust your carbohydrate intake. A healthcare professional can help you make these adjustments.

6. Plan meals ahead of time: Planning meals ahead of time can help you stay within your carbohydrate limits and ensure that you are getting balanced nutrition. A registered dietitian can help you develop a meal plan that is tailored to your individual needs.

7. Be mindful of portion sizes: Even healthy foods can lead to blood sugar spikes if consumed in large quantities. Be sure to pay attention to portion sizes and avoid overeating.

8. Consider the glycemic index: The glycemic index is a measure of how quickly a food raises blood sugar levels. Foods with a high glycemic index, such as white bread and sugary drinks, can cause blood sugar spikes. Choosing foods with a lower glycemic index, such as whole grains and non-starchy vegetables, can help to promote better blood sugar control.

9. Don't forget about drinks: Many drinks, such as fruit juice and soda, contain a high amount of carbohydrates. Be sure to factor in the carbohydrate content of your drinks when calculating your daily intake.

In addition to monitoring carbohydrate intake, it is also important to pay attention to the quality of the carbohydrates you consume. As discussed earlier, choosing complex carbohydrates and fiber-rich foods can help to promote better blood sugar control and reduce the risk of complications.

5

Making Healthy Food Choices

- **The importance of a balanced diet**

Maintaining a balanced and nutritious diet is essential for people with diabetes to manage their blood sugar levels and prevent complications. A balanced diet includes a variety of foods from all food groups, including:

1. Fruits and vegetables: These are rich in vitamins, minerals, and fiber, and can help to promote better blood sugar control. Aim for at least 5 servings of fruits and vegetables per day.
2. Whole grains: Whole grains, such as brown rice, quinoa, and whole wheat bread, are high in fiber and can help to slow the absorption of carbohydrates into the bloodstream.
3. Lean proteins: Choose lean sources of protein, such as chicken, fish, tofu, and legumes, to help build and repair body tissues.
4. Low-fat dairy: Low-fat dairy products, such as milk and yogurt, are rich in calcium and vitamin D, and can help to promote bone health.
5. Healthy fats: Include healthy fats, such as olive oil, avocado, and nuts, in your diet in moderation.
6. Reading food labels: Reading food labels can help you make informed choices about

the foods you eat. Pay attention to the serving size, total carbohydrate content, and added sugar content when selecting foods.

7. Eating mindfully: Eating mindfully involves paying attention to your food and the experience of eating. This can help you to avoid overeating and make healthier food choices.

8. Limiting alcohol intake: Alcohol can cause fluctuations in blood sugar levels and should be consumed in moderation or avoided altogether.

9. Staying hydrated: Drinking plenty of water is important for overall health and can also help to promote better blood sugar control.

In addition to choosing nutrient-rich foods, it is also important to pay attention to portion sizes and limit the intake of processed and high-sugar foods. Working with a registered dietitian can help you develop a meal plan that is tailored to your individual needs and preferences.

By following a balanced and nutritious diet, people with diabetes can improve their overall health and reduce the risk of complications.

- **Foods to eat and foods to avoid**

When managing diabetes through nutrition, it is important to make informed choices about the foods you eat. Some foods can help to promote better blood sugar control, while others can cause spikes in blood sugar levels and should be limited or avoided altogether.
Foods to Eat:

1. Non-starchy vegetables: Non-starchy vegetables, such as spinach, broccoli, and peppers, are low in calories and carbohydrates, and are rich in vitamins and minerals.
2. Whole grains: Whole grains, such as brown rice, quinoa, and whole wheat bread, are high in fiber and can help to slow the absorption of carbohydrates into the bloodstream.
3. Lean proteins: Choose lean sources of protein, such as chicken, fish, tofu, and legumes, to help build and repair body tissues.

4. Healthy fats: Include healthy fats, such as olive oil, avocado, and nuts, in your diet in moderation.
5. Low-fat dairy: Low-fat dairy products, such as milk and yogurt, are rich in calcium and vitamin D, and can help to promote bone health.
6. Fruits: Fruits are a good source of vitamins, minerals, and fiber, but should be eaten in moderation due to their natural sugar content.

Foods to Avoid:

1. Processed and high-sugar foods: Processed foods, such as candy, chips, and baked goods, are often high in sugar and can cause spikes in blood sugar levels.
2. Sugary drinks: Sugary drinks, such as soda and juice, are high in sugar and can cause fluctuations in blood sugar levels.
3. Trans and saturated fats: Trans and saturated fats, found in fried foods and high-fat dairy products, can increase the risk of heart disease and should be limited.

4. Refined carbohydrates: Refined carbohydrates, found in white bread, pasta, and rice, can cause spikes in blood sugar levels and should be limited.

By making informed choices about the foods you eat, people with diabetes can manage their blood sugar levels and reduce the risk of complications associated with the disease. It is important to work with a registered dietitian to develop a personalized nutrition plan that meets your individual needs and goals.

In addition to making healthy food choices, portion control is also an important aspect of managing diabetes through nutrition. Eating too much of any type of food, even healthy foods, can cause blood sugar levels to rise. It is recommended to use measuring cups, food scales, or other tools to help with portion control.

It is also important to pay attention to the timing and frequency of meals. Eating meals and snacks at regular intervals throughout the day can help to maintain stable blood sugar levels. Skipping meals or going too long without eating can cause blood sugar levels to drop too low, leading to symptoms such as dizziness, fatigue, and irritability.

In some cases, people with diabetes may benefit from following a specific diet plan, such as the Mediterranean diet or a low-carbohydrate diet. These diets have been shown to improve blood sugar control and reduce the risk of complications associated with diabetes. However, it is important to speak with a healthcare provider or registered dietitian before starting any new diet plan.

Overall, making healthy food choices and practicing portion control are essential components of managing diabetes through nutrition. By working with a healthcare team and making informed choices about the foods you eat, people with diabetes can improve their overall health and reduce the risk of complications associated with the disease.

- **Reading food labels**

Reading food labels is an important skill for people with diabetes who are managing their blood sugar levels through nutrition. Food labels provide information about the nutritional content of the food, including the total amount of carbohydrates, fats, and proteins in a serving size.

When reading food labels, it is important to pay attention to the serving size listed on the label. This will help to determine the amount of carbohydrates, fats, and proteins in a single serving. It is also important to look at the total number of carbohydrates listed, as well as the amount of sugar and fiber.

In general, people with diabetes should aim to choose foods that are low in sugar and high in fiber. This can help to prevent blood sugar spikes and promote feelings of fullness, which can help with portion control.

Food labels can also provide information about other important nutrients, such as vitamins and minerals. People with diabetes may need to pay special attention to certain nutrients, such as potassium and magnesium, which can help to lower blood pressure and improve overall health.

Overall, reading food labels is an important tool for people with diabetes who are managing their blood sugar levels through nutrition. By making informed choices about the foods they eat, people with diabetes can improve their overall health and reduce the risk of complications associated with the disease.

In addition to reading food labels, people with diabetes can benefit from learning about healthy meal planning strategies. This can include tips for creating balanced meals that incorporate a variety of different food groups, as well as guidelines for portion control and meal timing.

Some helpful tips for meal planning for people with diabetes include:

- Including a source of lean protein with each meal, such as skinless chicken breast, fish, tofu, or legumes
- Choosing low-carbohydrate vegetables, such as leafy greens, broccoli, and cauliflower, as the base of meals
- Limiting high-carbohydrate foods, such as bread, pasta, and rice, to smaller portions
- Incorporating healthy fats, such as nuts, seeds, avocado, and olive oil, in moderation

- Eating smaller, more frequent meals throughout the day to help stabilize blood sugar levels

By incorporating these strategies into their meal planning, people with diabetes can improve their blood sugar control and overall health. Additionally, working with a registered dietitian who specializes in diabetes nutrition can provide personalized support and guidance for developing a healthy meal plan that meets individual needs and preferences.

- **Sample meal plans**

Here are a few sample meal plans for people with diabetes:
1. Breakfast:
2 scrambled eggs
1 slice of whole-grain toast
1 small apple
Black coffee or tea with no sugar
Snack:
1 small low-fat yogurt
Lunch:
Grilled chicken breast

1/2 cup of brown rice

1 cup of steamed vegetables (broccoli, cauliflower, and carrots)

1 small orange

Snack:

1 small handful of almonds

Dinner:

Baked salmon fillet

1/2 cup of quinoa

1 cup of roasted vegetables (zucchini, bell peppers, and onions)

Small side salad with mixed greens, cucumber, and cherry tomatoes

1 small pear

sample meal plan

2. Breakfast:

1 cup of low-fat cottage cheese

1/2 cup of mixed berries (blueberries, raspberries, and strawberries)

1 slice of whole-grain toast with 1 teaspoon of peanut butter

Black coffee or tea with no sugar

Snack:

1 small apple

Lunch:

Tuna salad (1 can of tuna, mixed with 1 tablespoon of low-fat mayonnaise, diced celery, and onion)

1 small whole-grain pita bread

1 cup of sliced raw vegetables (carrots, cucumber, and cherry tomatoes)

1 small banana

Snack:

1 small low-fat yogurt

Dinner:

Grilled turkey breast

1/2 cup of quinoa

1 cup of steamed vegetables (asparagus, green beans, and mushrooms)

Small side salad with mixed greens, grated carrots, and sliced bell peppers

1 small orange

sample meal plan

3. Breakfast:

1/2 cup of oatmeal with 1/2 cup of mixed berries

1 small low-fat yogurt

Black coffee or tea with no sugar

Snack:

1 small handful of unsalted peanuts

Lunch:

Turkey and cheese sandwich (2 slices of whole-grain bread, 2 ounces of turkey breast, and 1 slice of low-fat cheese)

1 small apple

Small side salad with mixed greens and sliced cucumber

Snack:

1 small pear

Dinner:

Grilled fish fillet

1/2 cup of brown rice

1 cup of roasted vegetables (eggplant, zucchini, and onions)

Small side salad with mixed greens and sliced cherry tomatoes

1 small peach

It's important to note that these meal plans are just examples and should be adjusted to meet individual needs and preferences. A registered dietitian who specializes in diabetes nutrition can help develop a personalized meal plan that fits individual goals and lifestyles.

- **why these type of meal plans**

Sample meal plans can be helpful for people with diabetes who are struggling to create balanced meals that meet their nutritional needs. These meal plans are typically designed to provide a specific balance of carbohydrates, protein, and fat to help keep blood sugar levels stable throughout the day. They may also include recommendations for portion sizes and timing of meals and snacks.

Following a meal plan can also help people with diabetes to better understand how different foods affect their blood sugar levels, and can serve as a useful tool for making dietary adjustments if necessary. Additionally, meal plans can provide guidance and structure for people who are new to diabetes management or who may feel overwhelmed by the prospect of making dietary changes.

6

Managing Special Situations

- **Eating out with diabetes**

Managing diabetes while eating out can be challenging, but it is possible to make healthy choices and still enjoy a meal out. Here are some tips for eating out with diabetes:

1. Plan ahead: Look up the menu online before you go to the restaurant and decide what you will order ahead of time. This can help you avoid impulse decisions based on hunger or temptation.
2. Choose wisely: Look for menu items that are grilled, roasted, baked, or steamed rather than fried or sautéed. Choose dishes that are based on lean proteins such as fish, chicken, or tofu, and include plenty of non-starchy vegetables.
3. Watch portion sizes: Many restaurant meals are oversized, so be mindful of portion sizes and consider sharing a dish or taking leftovers home.
4. Be aware of hidden sugars: Many restaurant foods contain hidden sugars, such as in sauces, dressings, and marinades. Ask for these items on the side or choose dishes that are lower in added sugars.

5. Limit alcohol: Alcohol can cause blood sugar levels to fluctuate, so limit your intake or choose sugar-free mixers.
6. Speak up: Don't be afraid to ask your server questions about how a dish is prepared or for substitutions to make the meal healthier. Many restaurants are willing to accommodate special requests.
7. Be aware of timing: Try to time your meal so that it aligns with your medication or insulin regimen. For example, if you take insulin before meals, make sure your food arrives soon after you inject.
8. Bring your own snacks: If you're unsure about the options available or are worried about being hungry, bring along a healthy snack such as a piece of fruit or a handful of nuts.
9. Stay active: Eating out often means sitting for long periods of time, so make an effort to stay active throughout the day by taking a walk after your meal or choosing a restaurant that is within walking distance.

Remember, managing diabetes while eating out is all about making smart choices and being prepared. With a little planning, you can still enjoy a delicious meal out while keeping your blood sugar levels in check.

- **Managing diabetes during the holidays**

The holidays can be a challenging time for managing diabetes, with tempting treats and busy schedules. Here are some tips for staying on track during the holiday season:

1. Plan ahead: Look at your schedule and plan ahead for meals and snacks. Bring along healthy snacks to prevent yourself from indulging in unhealthy treats.
2. Be mindful of portion sizes: It's okay to indulge in your favorite holiday foods, but be mindful of portion sizes. Use a smaller plate and stick to one serving.
3. Be active: Make an effort to stay active during the holiday season. Take a walk after your meal or join in on a family activity.
4. Stick to your medication and insulin regimen: Don't skip or delay your medication or insulin injections, even if your schedule is busier than usual.

5. Communicate with family and friends: Let your family and friends know about your dietary needs and limitations. They may be willing to accommodate your needs or provide healthier options.

6. Watch your alcohol intake: Alcohol can affect blood sugar levels, so limit your intake and avoid sugary mixers.

7. Offer to bring a dish: If you're going to a holiday gathering, offer to bring a dish that fits within your dietary needs. This way, you know there will be at least one option that you can enjoy.

8. Modify recipes: Look for ways to modify traditional holiday recipes to make them healthier. For example, use sugar substitutes or reduce the amount of fat in a recipe.

9. Stay hydrated: Drinking plenty of water can help control blood sugar levels and keep you feeling full. Aim to drink at least eight glasses of water a day.

10. Take care of yourself: The holiday season can be stressful, so make sure to take care of yourself. Get plenty of sleep,

take time for yourself, and manage your stress levels.

Remember, the holidays are about spending time with loved ones and enjoying the season. With some planning and mindfulness, you can manage your diabetes while still enjoying the festivities.

- **Managing diabetes during pregnancy**

Managing diabetes during pregnancy is essential to ensure the health of both the mother and the baby. If you have gestational diabetes, your doctor will likely recommend a treatment plan that includes:

1. Monitoring blood sugar levels: You will need to monitor your blood sugar levels several times a day to ensure they are within a healthy range.
2. Healthy eating: Eating a balanced diet that is rich in nutrients and low in processed foods and added sugars is important for managing gestational diabetes.
3. Regular exercise: Exercise can help control blood sugar levels and promote a healthy

pregnancy. Your doctor can recommend safe exercises for you to do during pregnancy.

4. Medication: In some cases, your doctor may recommend medication, such as insulin, to help manage your blood sugar levels.

5. Regular prenatal care: Regular prenatal care is important for monitoring the health of both you and your baby. Your doctor will monitor your blood sugar levels, blood pressure, and other vital signs throughout your pregnancy.

6. Close monitoring after delivery: After delivery, your blood sugar levels will need to be closely monitored to ensure they return to normal.

By following these steps, you can help manage your gestational diabetes and ensure a healthy pregnancy and delivery. It's important to work closely with your healthcare team to create a treatment plan that meets your unique needs.

In addition to the above steps, it's important to be aware of the potential risks associated with gestational diabetes. These risks include:

1. High blood pressure: Women with gestational diabetes are at increased risk of developing high blood pressure during pregnancy.
2. Pre-eclampsia: Pre-eclampsia is a serious complication that can occur during pregnancy and is characterized by high blood pressure and damage to organs such as the liver and kidneys.
3. Preterm birth: Women with gestational diabetes are at increased risk of delivering their baby prematurely.
4. Large baby: Gestational diabetes can cause the baby to grow larger than usual, which can lead to difficulties during delivery.
5. Low blood sugar in the baby: After delivery, the baby may experience low blood sugar levels due to the mother's high blood sugar levels during pregnancy.

By being aware of these risks and following a comprehensive treatment plan, women with gestational diabetes can help ensure a healthy pregnancy and delivery. It's also important to talk to your healthcare provider about any concerns or questions you may have about managing diabetes during pregnancy.

Some additional tips for managing diabetes during pregnancy include:

1. Eating a healthy, balanced diet: A diet that is rich in whole grains, fruits, vegetables, lean protein, and healthy fats can help regulate blood sugar levels and provide essential nutrients for both the mother and the baby.

2. Staying physically active: Regular exercise can help regulate blood sugar levels and improve overall health during pregnancy. However, it's important to talk to your healthcare provider about what types of exercise are safe for you and your baby.

3. Monitoring blood sugar levels regularly: Pregnant women with diabetes may need to check their blood sugar levels more frequently than usual to ensure that they are within a healthy range.

4. Taking insulin as prescribed: If diet and exercise alone are not enough to regulate blood sugar levels, insulin injections may be necessary. It's important to take insulin as prescribed by your healthcare provider to ensure that blood sugar levels remain stable.
5. Attending regular prenatal checkups: Regular prenatal checkups are essential for monitoring the health of the mother and the baby and for identifying any potential complications early on.

By following these steps and working closely with your healthcare provider, it is possible to manage diabetes during pregnancy and ensure a healthy outcome for both the mother and the baby.

7

Benefits of Exercise

- **The importance of physical activity for people with diabetes**

Physical activity is crucial for people with diabetes. Regular exercise can help manage blood sugar levels by increasing the body's sensitivity to insulin, which helps the cells to use glucose for energy. Exercise also helps to reduce insulin resistance and lowers the risk of complications associated with diabetes, such as heart disease and stroke.

In addition, exercise can help improve overall health and well-being by reducing stress levels, improving circulation, strengthening muscles and bones, and helping to maintain a healthy weight.

The American Diabetes Association recommends at least 150 minutes of moderate-intensity aerobic exercise per week, spread out over at least three days per week, with no more than two consecutive days without exercise. It's also recommended to do strength training exercises at least two days per week, focusing on all major muscle groups.

It's important for people with diabetes to talk to their healthcare provider before starting any new exercise program to determine the safest and most effective activities for their individual needs.

Regular physical activity is crucial for everyone, especially for those with diabetes. Exercise offers a range of benefits that can help improve blood sugar control, reduce the risk of complications, and enhance overall health and well-being. Some of the benefits of exercise for people with diabetes include:

1. Improved blood sugar control: Exercise can help lower blood sugar levels by increasing insulin sensitivity and glucose uptake by muscles.
2. Weight management: Regular exercise can help manage body weight by burning

excess calories and increasing lean muscle mass.

3. Reduced risk of cardiovascular disease: Exercise can help improve cardiovascular health by reducing blood pressure, increasing HDL (good) cholesterol levels, and lowering LDL (bad) cholesterol levels.

4. Improved mental health: Exercise can help reduce stress and anxiety, enhance mood, and improve overall mental health.

5. Increased energy levels: Regular physical activity can increase energy levels and reduce fatigue, making it easier to perform daily activities.

6. Reduced risk of other chronic diseases: Exercise can help reduce the risk of other chronic diseases such as cancer, osteoporosis, and depression.

In short, exercise is an essential component of diabetes management and can offer numerous health benefits.

Regular physical activity offers numerous benefits for people with diabetes. It helps to:

1. Control blood sugar levels: Exercise helps to lower blood sugar levels by allowing muscles to use glucose for energy, even without insulin.
2. Improve insulin sensitivity: Regular physical activity helps your body to become more sensitive to insulin, allowing it to use insulin more effectively to move glucose from the bloodstream into the cells.
3. Control weight: Exercise burns calories, which helps to manage body weight. Maintaining a healthy weight can help to prevent and manage diabetes.
4. Reduce the risk of complications: Regular exercise can help to reduce the risk of diabetes-related complications, such as heart disease, stroke, and nerve damage.
5. Improve cardiovascular health: Exercise helps to strengthen the heart and improve blood flow, reducing the risk of heart disease, which is a common complication of diabetes.
6. Reduce stress: Exercise can help to reduce stress and anxiety, which can affect blood sugar levels.

7. Boost energy levels: Exercise helps to improve stamina and energy levels, making it easier to perform daily activities.
8. Improve overall health: Regular physical activity can help to improve overall health and well-being, including mental health.

Overall, incorporating regular physical activity into your diabetes management plan can have significant benefits for your health and quality of life.

- **Types of exercise (aerobic, strength training, flexibility)**

There are three main types of exercise that can benefit people with diabetes:

1. Aerobic Exercise: This type of exercise, also known as cardio or endurance exercise, involves continuous movement of large muscles in the arms, legs, and hips. Examples include brisk walking, jogging, cycling, swimming, dancing, and hiking. Aerobic exercise helps to improve cardiovascular health, lower blood glucose levels, and increase insulin sensitivity.

2. Strength Training: Also called resistance training, this type of exercise involves the use of weights, resistance bands, or bodyweight to build muscle and strength. Examples include weightlifting, push-ups, squats, lunges, and other resistance exercises. Strength training can help to increase muscle mass, improve glucose uptake by muscles, and increase insulin sensitivity.

3. Flexibility Exercise: This type of exercise involves stretching and improving the range of motion in the joints. Examples include yoga, Pilates, and stretching exercises. Flexibility exercise can help to improve balance, reduce the risk of falls, and reduce stress levels.

All three types of exercise are important for people with diabetes, and a combination of aerobic, strength training, and flexibility exercises can provide the most benefit.

Aerobic exercise, also known as cardio exercise, involves activities that increase your heart rate and breathing rate, such as walking, running, cycling, swimming, and dancing.

This type of exercise can help improve your cardiovascular health, lower your blood pressure and cholesterol levels, and increase your body's sensitivity to insulin.

Strength training, also known as resistance training, involves using weights, resistance bands, or body weight exercises to build muscle mass and strength. This type of exercise can help improve your glucose control by increasing insulin sensitivity, as well as improving your bone density and reducing the risk of falls and fractures.

Flexibility exercises, such as stretching and yoga, can help improve your range of motion and reduce the risk of injury during exercise. They can also help reduce stress and promote relaxation, which can be beneficial for managing diabetes.

It's important to note that before starting an exercise program, it's important to speak with your healthcare provider to ensure that it's safe for you to do so, and to determine what types and amount of exercise are appropriate for your individual needs and abilities.

- **Safe exercise guidelines for people with diabetes**

Safe exercise guidelines for people with diabetes include:

1. Consult your doctor before starting any exercise program: People with diabetes have varying levels of physical ability and medical history, so it is essential to consult a doctor before starting any exercise program.
2. Start slowly and gradually increase intensity: People with diabetes should start with light or moderate exercise and gradually increase the intensity as they become more comfortable with the activity.
3. Choose low-impact activities: Low-impact activities such as swimming, walking, cycling, and yoga are excellent options for people with diabetes. These activities are easy on the joints and can help improve cardiovascular health.
4. Monitor blood glucose levels: People with diabetes should monitor their blood glucose levels before, during, and after exercise. If

blood glucose levels are too low or too high, exercise should be avoided.

5. Stay hydrated: Drinking water before, during, and after exercise is essential to keep the body hydrated and to prevent dehydration.

6. Wear appropriate footwear: Wearing proper footwear can prevent foot injuries and help maintain balance during exercise.

7. Carry a source of carbohydrates: People with diabetes should always carry a source of carbohydrates such as juice or glucose tablets in case of low blood sugar during exercise.

8. Stop exercising if you experience any symptoms: If you experience symptoms such as dizziness, chest pain, or shortness of breath, stop exercising and seek medical attention immediately.

8

Incorporating Exercise into Your Routine

- ## How to start an exercise program

Starting an exercise program can seem intimidating, but it is important to remember that any physical activity is better than none. Here are some tips to help you get started:

1. Consult your healthcare team: Before starting an exercise program, it is important to talk to your healthcare team. They can help you determine what type of exercise is best for you and what level of intensity is safe.

2. Set realistic goals: Start with small, achievable goals that you can gradually build upon. For example, aim to walk for 10 minutes a day and gradually increase to 30 minutes.

3. Choose activities you enjoy: You are more likely to stick to an exercise program if you

enjoy the activities. Try different types of exercise until you find something that you like.

4. Make it a habit: Schedule your exercise like you would any other appointment. Consistency is key when it comes to exercise.
5. Start slowly: Begin with low-intensity activities and gradually increase the duration and intensity over time.
6. Monitor your blood sugar levels: Exercise can affect your blood sugar levels, so it is important to monitor them before, during, and after exercise.
7. Stay hydrated: Drink plenty of water before, during, and after exercise.
8. Wear appropriate shoes and clothing: Choose comfortable, supportive shoes and clothing that allows for movement.
9. Warm-up and cool down: Always warm up before exercising and cool down afterward to prevent injury.

Remember, it's important to listen to your body and adjust your exercise routine as needed. If you experience any pain or discomfort, stop exercising and talk to your healthcare team.

- **Tips for staying motivated**

Here are some tips for staying motivated to exercise:

1. Set achievable goals: Setting achievable goals is important because it helps you stay motivated. Start with small goals and gradually increase the intensity and duration of your exercise routine.
2. Find an exercise buddy: Exercising with a friend or family member can make it more enjoyable and can help you stay motivated.
3. Mix it up: Doing the same exercise routine every day can get boring, so try different types of exercises to keep it interesting.
4. Reward yourself: Set up a reward system for yourself when you reach a specific goal. This can be a great motivator to keep going.
5. Schedule your workouts: Make exercise a part of your daily routine and schedule it into your calendar.
6. Track your progress: Tracking your progress can help you see how far you've

come and give you a sense of accomplishment.

7. Focus on the benefits: Remind yourself of the benefits of exercise, such as improved blood sugar control, weight loss, increased energy, and improved mood.

Remember, it's important to find activities you enjoy and that fit into your lifestyle to help you stay motivated and make exercise a regular part of your routine.

- **Exercise safety tips for people with diabetes**

Exercise can have many benefits for people with diabetes, but it's important to take some precautions to exercise safely. Here are some exercise safety tips for people with diabetes:

1. Check with your doctor: Before starting an exercise program, it's important to get your doctor's approval, especially if you have any complications from diabetes or other health issues.

2. Monitor your blood sugar: Check your blood sugar before, during, and after

exercise to make sure it stays within a safe range. If your blood sugar is too low or too high, it can be dangerous to exercise.

3. Have a snack: If your blood sugar is low before exercising, have a small snack, such as a piece of fruit or a granola bar, to raise your blood sugar.

4. Stay hydrated: Drink plenty of water before, during, and after exercise to stay hydrated. Dehydration can cause your blood sugar to rise.

5. Wear proper footwear: Wear well-fitting, comfortable shoes that provide good support to prevent foot injuries.

6. Avoid exercising in extreme temperatures: Hot or cold temperatures can affect your blood sugar, so try to exercise indoors or during mild weather conditions.

7. Carry identification: Always carry identification that indicates you have diabetes, in case of an emergency.

8. Start slowly: Begin with short, easy exercises and gradually increase the intensity and duration as your fitness level improves.

Remember, exercise can be an important part of diabetes management, but it's important to exercise safely and consult with your doctor before starting any exercise program.

9

Coping with the Emotional Impact of Diabetes

- **The emotional impact of diabetes**

Living with diabetes can be emotionally challenging. It is normal to experience a wide range of emotions, including fear, anger, sadness, frustration, and guilt. Coping with the emotional impact of diabetes is just as important as managing your blood sugar levels.

Here are some practical tips for coping with the emotional impact of diabetes:

1. Seek support: Talk to your friends, family, or a therapist about how you're feeling. Joining a support group can also be helpful.
2. Educate yourself: Learn as much as you can about diabetes. Knowledge is power, and the more you know, the better equipped you will be to manage your diabetes.
3. Stay positive: Focus on what you can do to manage your diabetes, rather than on what you can't do. Celebrate your successes, no matter how small.
4. Practice self-care: Take care of yourself physically and emotionally. Make time for activities that you enjoy, such as hobbies, exercise, or spending time with loved ones.
5. Manage stress: Stress can affect blood sugar levels, so it's important to manage it. Try relaxation techniques, such as deep breathing or meditation.
6. Set realistic goals: Break your goals down into smaller, more manageable steps. Celebrate your progress along the way.

Remember, it's normal to experience a range of emotions when living with diabetes. Don't be afraid to ask for help or support when you need it.

Being diagnosed with diabetes can be a life-changing experience that can lead to emotional and psychological distress. The emotional impact of diabetes can be different for each individual and may include feelings of anxiety, depression, anger, denial, guilt, and frustration. Diabetes requires significant lifestyle changes, and the need to manage the condition can be overwhelming and stressful.

The stress of managing diabetes can affect not only the person with the condition but also their family and loved ones. It is important to recognize the emotional impact of diabetes and to seek support to help manage these feelings. Counseling, support groups, and talking to friends and family can all be helpful in coping with the emotional impact of diabetes.

Living with diabetes can be emotionally challenging for many individuals, as it requires constant attention to blood sugar levels, food choices, and medication management. Diabetes can also impact one's self-image, relationships, and overall quality of life. Some people may experience feelings of anger, frustration, guilt, anxiety, or depression related to their diabetes diagnosis.

The emotional impact of diabetes can also affect one's ability to manage the condition effectively. Stress and negative emotions can raise blood sugar levels, making it harder to achieve target levels. Conversely, a positive outlook and strong emotional support system can help individuals manage their diabetes more effectively.

It's essential to address the emotional impact of diabetes and seek support when needed. This may include talking to a healthcare provider, joining a support group, or seeking the help of a mental health professional. By taking care of emotional health, individuals with diabetes can improve their overall well-being and manage the condition more effectively.

- **Strategies for coping with diabetes-related stress and anxiety**

Managing diabetes can be a stressful and overwhelming experience for many people. It is normal to feel frustrated, anxious, and depressed about the challenges that come with managing this chronic condition. However, it is important to find healthy ways to cope with these emotions and reduce stress to maintain good physical and emotional health. Here are some strategies for coping with diabetes-related stress and anxiety:

1. Stay connected: Reach out to family, friends, or a support group to share your feelings and experiences. Talking about your concerns can help you feel less alone and more supported.
2. Practice relaxation techniques: Techniques such as deep breathing, meditation, and yoga can help reduce stress and promote relaxation.
3. Stay active: Exercise is not only good for your physical health but can also boost your mood and help manage stress.
4. Set achievable goals: Break down larger goals into smaller, achievable ones. This can help you feel more in control of your

diabetes management and reduce feelings of overwhelm.

5. Seek professional help: If you are struggling with your emotions, it is important to seek professional help. Consider talking to a mental health professional who can help you develop coping strategies and provide additional support.

6. Stay positive: Focus on the positive aspects of your life and your diabetes management. Celebrate your successes and remember that setbacks are a normal part of the process.

Remember that managing diabetes is a journey, and it is normal to experience a range of emotions along the way. By finding healthy ways to cope with stress and anxiety, you can improve your overall well-being and make the most out of your diabetes management.

Here are some additional strategies for coping with diabetes-related stress and anxiety:

1. Practice relaxation techniques: Engage in activities that help to calm your mind and body, such as deep breathing, meditation, or yoga. These techniques can help to reduce stress and anxiety levels.

2. Seek support: It can be helpful to talk to others who have diabetes and understand what you're going through. Joining a support group or speaking with a counselor can also provide a safe space to express your feelings and concerns.

3. Stay organized: Diabetes management can be overwhelming, but staying organized can help to reduce stress levels. Keep track of your medications, blood sugar levels, and appointments in a journal or planner.

4. Focus on the positives: While diabetes can be challenging, it's important to focus on the positives and celebrate small victories. This can help to boost your mood and motivation.

5. Practice self-care: Taking care of yourself physically, mentally, and emotionally is essential for managing diabetes. This includes getting enough sleep, eating a healthy diet, exercising regularly, and

engaging in activities that bring you joy and relaxation.

- **The importance of social support**

Social support can play a significant role in helping people with diabetes manage their condition. Support from family, friends, and healthcare professionals can provide encouragement, accountability, and practical assistance. Support groups can also be a valuable resource, providing a forum for people with diabetes to share experiences, advice, and emotional support.

Having a support system can help people with diabetes adhere to their treatment plan and make lifestyle changes, such as eating healthy and exercising regularly. It can also reduce feelings of isolation and provide a sense of community.

It's important for people with diabetes to communicate their needs to their support system, whether it's help with meal planning, emotional support, or encouragement to exercise. With the right support, people with diabetes can successfully manage their condition and improve their quality of life.

10

Traveling with Diabetes

- **Preparing for travel with diabetes**

Traveling with diabetes can require some extra planning and preparation to ensure that you have everything you need to manage your diabetes while on the go. Here are some tips for preparing for travel with diabetes:

1. Consult with your healthcare provider: Before you travel, schedule an appointment

with your healthcare provider to discuss your travel plans. They can provide you with specific advice on how to manage your diabetes while traveling and can help you make any necessary adjustments to your medication or insulin regimen.

2. Pack extra supplies: Be sure to pack more than enough diabetes supplies for your trip, including insulin, syringes or pens, glucose meter, test strips, lancets, and batteries. Pack these supplies in your carry-on luggage so that you have them with you at all times.

3. Bring a doctor's note: If you are traveling internationally, it may be helpful to bring a letter from your doctor explaining that you have diabetes and need to carry diabetes supplies with you.

4. Plan for time zone changes: If you are traveling to a different time zone, talk to your healthcare provider about how to adjust your insulin regimen to account for the time difference.

5. Check with your airline: If you are flying, check with your airline to see if they have any specific rules or regulations regarding

diabetes supplies. You may need to carry a doctor's note or obtain special permission to bring your supplies on board.

6. Research local food options: Before you travel, research local food options and familiarize yourself with the carbohydrate content of typical meals. This can help you make healthy food choices while on the go.

7. Carry snacks: Be sure to carry snacks with you, such as granola bars or fruit, to help keep your blood sugar levels stable while traveling.

8. Stay hydrated: Drink plenty of water while traveling to prevent dehydration, which can affect your blood sugar levels.

9. Be prepared for emergencies: Carry a glucagon kit with you in case of an emergency. Make sure that your travel companions are aware of your diabetes and know how to administer glucagon if necessary.

10. Stay in touch with your healthcare provider: If you experience any problems managing your diabetes while traveling, contact your healthcare provider for guidance and support.

- **Tips for managing diabetes while traveling**

Here are some tips for managing diabetes while traveling:

1. Plan ahead: Make sure to pack all necessary supplies, including medications, glucose testing strips, lancets, and insulin, as well as snacks and other emergency supplies.
2. Keep medication and supplies with you: Pack all medications and supplies in your carry-on luggage or personal item. Never check them with your luggage, in case it gets lost or delayed.
3. Adjust for time zone changes: If you are traveling across time zones, talk to your doctor about how to adjust your medication schedule accordingly.
4. Be aware of changes in diet: If you are traveling to a new country, be aware of changes in the diet and how they may affect your blood sugar levels. Pack snacks that you know are safe and healthy for you.

5. Stay hydrated: Drink plenty of water while traveling, as dehydration can affect blood sugar levels.
6. Check blood sugar levels regularly: Check your blood sugar levels regularly, especially if you are experiencing changes in routine or diet.
7. Carry identification: Wear a medical alert bracelet or necklace that identifies you as a person with diabetes, in case of emergency.
8. Inform travel companions: Inform your travel companions about your diabetes, and how they can help you in case of emergency.
9. Know local medical resources: Look up local medical resources, such as hospitals and clinics, in case of emergency.

By following these tips, you can manage your diabetes while traveling and enjoy your trip with peace of mind.

- **What to pack for travel**

When traveling with diabetes, it's important to pack all the necessary items to manage your condition. Here are some things to consider bringing:

1. Medications: Make sure to pack enough insulin and other diabetes medications to last the duration of your trip. It's also a good idea to bring a backup supply in case of emergency.
2. Glucose meter and supplies: Bring your glucose meter, test strips, and lancets. Also, consider packing extra batteries and a charger for your meter.
3. Snacks: Bring healthy snacks such as nuts, fruit, and granola bars in case you need to eat in between meals.
4. Water bottle: Staying hydrated is important for managing blood sugar levels. Bring a reusable water bottle to fill up throughout the day.
5. Medical ID bracelet: A medical ID bracelet or necklace can help emergency responders identify that you have diabetes and provide appropriate care.
6. Doctor's note: If you're traveling with insulin or other medications, it's a good

idea to bring a doctor's note explaining your condition and medications.

7. Travel cooler: If you're traveling with insulin that needs to be refrigerated, consider bringing a travel cooler to keep it at the proper temperature.
8. Contact information: Bring contact information for your doctor and diabetes care team in case you need to reach them while traveling.
9. Travel insurance: Consider purchasing travel insurance that includes coverage for diabetes-related care in case of an emergency.

When packing for travel, people with diabetes need to ensure they have enough supplies to manage their condition throughout their trip. It is recommended to pack at least twice as many supplies as you think you will need, just in case of unexpected delays or losses. Some essential items to pack include:

1. Insulin and medications: Pack enough insulin and medications to last throughout

the trip, as well as extras in case of emergency.

2. Blood glucose monitoring supplies: Pack your glucose meter, extra batteries, lancets, test strips, and any other supplies needed to check your blood glucose levels.

3. Snacks: Pack healthy snacks, such as nuts, fruit, and whole-grain crackers, to keep blood sugar levels stable while traveling.

4. Medical identification: Wear a medical alert bracelet or necklace that identifies you as having diabetes, in case of a medical emergency.

5. Doctor's letter: Bring a letter from your doctor that outlines your diabetes treatment plan and lists all the medications you take, including insulin.

6. Cooler bag: Bring a cooler bag to keep insulin and other medications cool during travel.

7. Travel insurance: Consider purchasing travel insurance that covers any diabetes-related emergencies, such as hospitalization or the need for medical evacuation.

It's also important to research your destination and find out what resources are available for people with diabetes. For example, some countries may have different types of insulin that require different dosages or injection techniques. Knowing this information ahead of time can help prevent any complications while traveling.

11

Managing Medications and Medical Appointments

- **Importance of medication adherence**

Medication adherence is crucial for managing diabetes effectively. Diabetes medications help lower blood sugar levels, which can prevent or delay complications from diabetes. It is essential to take the prescribed medications as directed by the healthcare provider to prevent fluctuations in blood sugar levels.

Skipping doses or taking medication at the wrong time can lead to unstable blood sugar levels, which can be dangerous for people with diabetes. It is essential to communicate with the healthcare provider about any difficulties or concerns related to medication management to ensure that the treatment plan is tailored to the individual's needs.

It is also essential to keep an up-to-date record of medications, dosages, and schedules to avoid any confusion or errors. Using a pill organizer or medication reminder apps can help ensure medication adherence.

Regular medical appointments are crucial for monitoring diabetes control and addressing any health concerns. The healthcare provider may adjust the treatment plan based on the individual's needs and blood sugar levels. It is essential to attend all scheduled appointments and communicate any issues or concerns with the healthcare provider.

- **Understanding your medications**

Understanding your medications is crucial for managing your diabetes effectively. It's important to know what your medications do, when to take them, and any potential side effects. Your healthcare provider or pharmacist can help you understand your medications and answer any questions you may have. Some common medications used to manage diabetes include:

1. Insulin: Insulin is a hormone that helps regulate blood sugar levels. It's usually injected under the skin using a syringe or insulin pen. There are several types of insulin available, including rapid-acting, short-acting, intermediate-acting, and long-acting.
2. Metformin: Metformin is an oral medication that helps lower blood sugar

levels by decreasing the amount of glucose produced by the liver.

3. Sulfonylureas: Sulfonylureas are oral medications that stimulate the pancreas to release more insulin.

4. GLP-1 receptor agonists: GLP-1 receptor agonists are injectable medications that help regulate blood sugar levels by increasing insulin production and decreasing the amount of glucose produced by the liver.

5. DPP-4 inhibitors: DPP-4 inhibitors are oral medications that help regulate blood sugar levels by increasing insulin production and decreasing the amount of glucose produced by the liver.

6. SGLT2 inhibitors: SGLT2 inhibitors are oral medications that help regulate blood sugar levels by increasing glucose excretion through the urine.

It's important to take your medications as prescribed and to let your healthcare provider know if you experience any side effects or have difficulty adhering to your medication regimen.

Understanding your medications involves knowing the purpose, dosage, frequency, and side effects of each medication. It is important to understand how your medications work to manage your diabetes and to follow your healthcare provider's instructions for taking them.

Your healthcare provider may prescribe different types of medications, such as insulin, oral medications, or a combination of both. Each medication has a specific purpose and works differently in the body. It is important to know when and how to take each medication and to monitor your blood sugar levels regularly to ensure that they are working effectively.

If you have any questions or concerns about your medications, it is important to discuss them with your healthcare provider. They can provide you with detailed information about your medications and address any concerns you may have.

It is also important to keep track of your medications and to refill them before they run out. This helps ensure that you do not miss any doses and that you have enough medication on hand for emergencies.

In addition to taking your medications as prescribed, it is important to keep up with your medical appointments. This includes regular check-ups with your healthcare provider, as well as appointments with any specialists, such as a diabetes educator or endocrinologist.

During these appointments, your healthcare provider can monitor your blood sugar levels, review your medications, and make any necessary adjustments to your treatment plan. They can also provide guidance and support for managing your diabetes and making healthy lifestyle choices.

- **Keeping track of medical appointments**

Keeping track of medical appointments is an essential aspect of diabetes management. It is important to schedule and attend regular appointments with healthcare professionals, including primary care physicians, endocrinologists, ophthalmologists, and podiatrists. These appointments are crucial for monitoring and managing diabetes-related complications and ensuring that diabetes is well-controlled.

There are several ways to keep track of medical appointments:

1. Use a calendar: Mark your medical appointments on a calendar or planner to keep track of the dates and times. This will help you avoid scheduling conflicts and ensure that you don't miss any appointments.
2. Set reminders: Use a reminder app on your phone or computer to alert you of upcoming appointments. This will help you stay on top of your schedule and ensure that you are prepared for each appointment.
3. Keep a medical diary: Record your medical appointments, test results, and medications in a medical diary or journal. This will help you keep track of your progress and ensure that you are receiving the appropriate treatment.
4. Use technology: Many healthcare providers offer online portals or apps that allow patients to schedule appointments, access

medical records, and receive appointment reminders.

By staying organized and keeping track of medical appointments, you can ensure that you receive the best possible care and manage your diabetes effectively.

Keeping track of medical appointments is an essential aspect of diabetes management. It is recommended to see your doctor at least every three to six months to monitor your blood sugar levels and adjust your treatment plan if necessary.

To keep track of your medical appointments, you can use a variety of tools such as a calendar, a planner, or a diabetes management app. Some apps are specifically designed to help you manage your diabetes, track your blood sugar levels, and schedule your appointments.

It is also important to prepare for your medical appointments by making a list of questions to ask your doctor and bringing along any relevant medical records or glucose monitoring logs. This can help ensure that you have a productive appointment and get the most out of your time with your healthcare provider.

If you have trouble remembering your appointments or have difficulty making it to them, you may want to consider setting reminders on your phone or asking a friend or family member to help you stay on track. With the right tools and support, managing your medical appointments can become an effortless part of your diabetes management routine.

12

Conclusion (Encouragement)

- **Recap of key takeaways**

In summary, here are some key takeaways from this guide on managing diabetes:

1. Diabetes can be effectively managed with a combination of medication, lifestyle changes, and self-monitoring of blood sugar levels.
2. Regular monitoring of blood sugar levels is crucial for managing diabetes, and there are different methods available for doing so, including self-monitoring and continuous glucose monitoring.
3. Understanding carbohydrates is important for managing blood sugar levels, and it is recommended to consume complex carbohydrates over simple ones.
4. Maintaining a balanced diet, reading food labels, and making healthy food choices are important strategies for managing diabetes.
5. Special situations such as eating out, holidays, and pregnancy require careful planning and management.
6. Exercise is an important part of diabetes management and can help improve blood

sugar control, cardiovascular health, and overall well-being.

7. Coping with the emotional impact of diabetes and having a support system are important for overall well-being.
8. Adhering to medication schedules and keeping track of medical appointments are essential for managing diabetes effectively.
9. With proper management, people with diabetes can lead healthy and fulfilling lives.

- **Resources for further reading**

Here are some resources for further reading on diabetes management:

1. American Diabetes Association (ADA) - https://www.diabetes.org/
2. Centers for Disease Control and Prevention (CDC) - https://www.cdc.gov/diabetes/index.html
3. National Institute of Diabetes and Digestive and Kidney Diseases (NIDDK) - https://www.niddk.nih.gov/health-information/diabetes

4. Mayo Clinic - https://www.mayoclinic.org/diseases-conditions/diabetes/symptoms-causes/syc-20371444
5. Diabetes Self-Management Magazine - https://www.diabetesselfmanagement.com/

These resources provide a wealth of information on managing diabetes, including advice on nutrition, exercise, medication, and other aspects of diabetes care. They also offer support and resources for individuals living with diabetes and their loved ones.

- **Encouragement to take control of your diabetes and live a healthy, fulfilling life.**

Great job! You now have a comprehensive guide to managing diabetes. Remember, taking control of your diabetes is a journey, not a destination. It takes time, effort, and patience to establish a routine that works for you. But with the right tools, support, and mindset, you can live a healthy, fulfilling life with diabetes. Don't be afraid to ask for help from healthcare professionals, loved ones, and diabetes support groups. Keep learning, stay motivated, and take action to manage your diabetes and live your best life.

.....***.....